MEAL PREP COOKBOOK

30-day meal plan with photos
easy and healthy meals to cook, prep,
grab and go

Table of Contents

—

3

Introduction

Why is this Meal Prep Cookbook release so important? Because at MEAL PREP, we believe in the power of preparing today's foods with the assurance that you'll always have healthy options to get the body and mind ready for tomorrow. This cookbook is full of easy recipes that will save you money and help you achieve your fitness goals.

In recent years, Meal Prep has become an emerging trend as people realize the benefits of spending time preparing meals in advance. Convenience, cost-effectiveness, and time-saving are the main factors contributing to the growing popularity of meal prep. If you are a busy working professional, meal prep will help you cut down on the money and time you spend on buying take-outs from the office cafeteria. It will also help you stay away from junk food and better control your caloric intake. Preparing a few portions of your favorite meals can help you save money and feel energetic enough to make it through the long and busy work schedule and daily responsibilities.

The most significant advantage of prepping your own meals is the chance to personalize your meals. This factor makes prepping meals more enjoyable and exciting. Individuals used to buy prepared meals from their local grocery stores and take their meals to work. It cost money and took up most of their time only to have it eaten in front of them while they are sitting at their desks all day.

While the benefits of meal prep can be split into two main categories: financial and health, it saves lots of your finances in the long run by reaping the benefits of cheaper food. You will also enjoy healthier eating because you already chose what and how much to eat. Not to mention, meal prep is an excellent way to stay consistent with your goals and objectives. For anyone who wants to lose weight, for example, the key to long-term success is consistency. To succeed with weight loss, you must stay in control of your diet. If you are going about it the right way and planning ahead, you will lose weight much easier than you ever thought possible.

It also allows you to eat healthy throughout the week without worrying about finding time to shop or cook. This meal prep cookbook includes a wide range of recipes so that you can use this book for multiple purposes. You can use these recipes for meal prepping, as well as making them from scratch for your family and friends.

How to Meal Prep?

There are different ways on how you can meal prep if you're a beginner in this journey. Some of them are the following:

Make-Ahead Meals

Prepare for the week ahead and freeze the meals that you plan to cook every week. This kind of meal preparation is easy and saves time in the summer. Using freezer containers is a great way to preserve food for future use. The frozen meals taste great and have fewer ingredients. You will also save your wallet on fresh groceries.

Batch Cooking

This meal prep method involves preparing multiple recipes at a time and cooking them all together. It is an excellent way to prepare several meals fast. This method's advantage is that it is economical since you can prepare large portions of food in one go.

Individually Portioned Meals

Prepare food individually and make sure they will be ready fast. This method is perfect for a week filled with celebrations. You can prepare each meal individually in the evening and enjoy the benefits of eating right out of the containers.

Ready-To-Cook Ingredients

If you're a busy person who does not have much time to cook in the morning, shopping for ready-to-cook ingredients will do. Buying and preparing fresh ingredients ahead of time will help you save time in the busy mornings. But make sure to eat fresh meals. As soon as the ingredients are bought, they will also spoil if not eaten straight away. Therefore, you need to plan your meals ahead of time to make sure you will use them before they get stale.

Now that you know the basics and advantages of meal prepping, it's time to get down to the most awaited 500 meal prep recipes with the 30-day meal plan by the end of it. We hope you'll enjoy the wide range of meals but make sure to make them in your own way. If you are a vegan, don't add meat to your recipes. If you are a vegetarian, add some meat to the recipe. Most importantly, don't fear to play around with your recipes! Happy meal prepping.

Breakfast

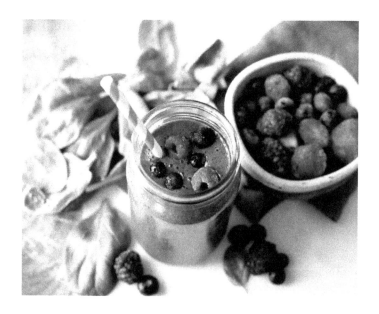

Spinach-Berry Smoothie Packs

Preparation time: 10 minutes

Cooking time: 0 minutes

Servings: 5

Ingredients:

- 10 cups baby spinach, washed and patted dry
- 2½ cups fresh or frozen strawberries
- 2½ cups fresh or frozen blueberries or blackberries
- 5 pitted dates
- 3¾ cups apple juice, divided

Directions:

1. Into each of 5 resealable plastic bags, put 2 cups of spinach, ½ cup of strawberries, ½ cup of blueberries, and 1 date. Seal the bags and freeze for at least 2 hours.
2. When ready to make the smoothie, pour ¾ cup of apple juice into the blender. Put the contents of one smoothie pack, then blend until smooth. Pour into a to-go cup and enjoy.

Nutrition:

Calories: 241

Fat: 0g

Protein: 3g

Carbs: 62g

Morning Sunshine Smoothie Packs

Preparation time: 15 minutes

Cooking time: 0 minutes

Servings: 5

Ingredients:

- 5 medium bananas, cut into chunks
- Zest of 1 orange, divided
- 5 medium carrots, shredded
- 2½ cups fresh sliced or frozen pineapple chunks
- 1 pitted date
- 3¾ cups nonfat milk, divided

Directions:

1. Into each of 5 resealable plastic bags, put chunks of 1 banana, about ½ teaspoon of orange zest, 1 shredded carrot, ½ cup of pineapple, and 1 date. Seal the bags and freeze for at least 2 hours.
2. When ready to make the smoothie, pour ¾ cup of milk into the blender. Put the contents of one smoothie pack, then blend until smooth. Pour into a to-go cup and enjoy.

Nutrition:

Calories: 252

Fat: 1g

Protein: 10g

Carbs: 55g

Blackberry Bran Muffins

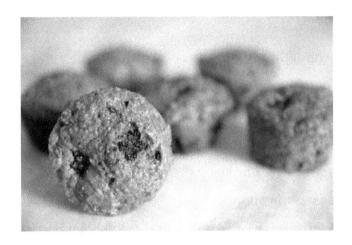

Preparation time: 15 minutes

Cooking time: 20 minutes

Servings: 12

Ingredients:

- Nonstick cooking spray
- 2 cups whole-wheat flour or white whole-wheat flour
- ¼ cup oat bran
- 2 teaspoons baking powder
- 1 teaspoon baking soda
- ¼ teaspoon salt
- ½ cup light brown sugar
- ½ cup low-fat (1%) milk
- ½ cup olive oil or canola oil
- 1 cup reduced-fat (2%) plain Greek yogurt
- 1 large egg + 1 large egg yolk
- 1 teaspoon vanilla extract
- 1½ cups fresh or frozen and thawed blackberries
- ¼ cup rolled oats, divided

Directions:

1. Preheat the oven to 375F. Coat a 12-muffin tin with cooking spray and set aside. In a medium bowl, sift the flour, oat bran, baking powder, baking soda, and salt.
2. Whisk the brown sugar, milk, and oil in a large bowl. Add the yogurt, egg, egg yolk, and vanilla. Whisk until smooth.

3. Gently fold the dry fixings into the wet ingredients, being careful not to overmix. Gently fold in the blackberries to evenly distribute them throughout the batter.
4. Using a ¼-cup scoop, transfer the batter into the prepared muffin tin. Tap it a few times on your counter to remove any air bubbles.
5. Sprinkle each muffin using 1 teaspoon of rolled oats. Bake within 20 minutes until golden brown and a toothpick inserted in the center comes out clean.
6. Remove, then allow to cool within 10 minutes before removing the muffins from the tin.

Nutrition:

Calories: 217

Fat: 11g

Protein: 7g

Carbs: 26g

Pear–Pumpkin Seed Muffins

Preparation time: 15 minutes

Cooking time: 22 minutes

Servings: 12

Ingredients:

- Nonstick cooking spray
- 1¼ cups unbleached all-purpose flour
- 1 cup whole-wheat pastry flour
- 1 teaspoon baking powder
- ½ teaspoon baking soda
- 1/8 teaspoon salt
- ½ cup creamy almond/sunflower seed butter, at room temperature
- ½ cup nonfat plain Greek yogurt
- ½ cup low-fat (1%) milk
- ½ cup packed light brown sugar
- ½ cup applesauce
- 1/3 cup canola oil
- 2 large eggs
- 1 teaspoon vanilla extract
- 1 medium pear, diced
- ½ cup unsalted roasted pumpkin seeds, divided

Directions:

1. Preheat the oven to 350F. Coat a 12-cup muffin tin using cooking spray, then set aside. In a medium bowl, sift the all-purpose flour, pastry flour, baking powder, baking soda, plus salt.
2. Whisk the almond butter, yogurt, plus milk until smooth in a large bowl. Put the brown sugar, applesauce, plus oil, then stir until combined. Put the eggs, one at a time, then the vanilla, stirring until completely incorporated.
3. Fold the dry fixing into the wet ingredients, and stir until just blended, careful not to overmix. Gently fold in the pear and ¼ cup of pumpkin seeds.
4. Using a ¼-cup scoop, distribute the batter among the prepared muffin cups. Tap it a few times on your counter to remove any air bubbles. Sprinkle each muffin cup with 1 tsp of pumpkin seeds.
5. Bake within 22 minutes until the tops are browned. Remove, and allow to cool within 10 minutes before removing the muffins from the tin.

Nutrition:

Calories: 296

Fat: 15g

Protein: 9g

Carbs: 33g

Pumpkin Breakfast Blondies

Preparation time: 15 minutes

Cooking time: 20 minutes

Servings: 15

Ingredients:

- Nonstick cooking spray
- 1¼ cups whole-wheat flour or white whole-wheat flour
- 1½ cups rolled oats
- 1 teaspoon ground cinnamon
- ½ teaspoon baking soda
- ¼ teaspoon salt
- ¼ teaspoon ground ginger
- ¼ teaspoon ground allspice
- 1/8 teaspoon ground cloves
- 1/8 teaspoon ground nutmeg
- 2 tablespoons unsalted butter, melted
- ¼ cup nonfat plain Greek yogurt
- ½ cup 100% pure maple syrup
- ¼ cup light brown sugar
- ½ cup pumpkin purée
- 1 large egg
- 1 teaspoon vanilla extract

Directions:

1. Preheat the oven to 350F. Coat an 8-by-11.5-inch or similar size baking pan with cooking spray. Sift the flour, oats, cinnamon, baking soda, salt, ginger, allspice, cloves, and nutmeg in a medium bowl.
2. Whisk the butter, yogurt, maple syrup, and brown sugar in a large bowl. Add the pumpkin purée, egg, and vanilla, whisking until smooth.
3. Gently fold the dry fixings into the wet ingredients until thoroughly blended.
4. Put the batter into your prepared pan, then use a spatula to distribute evenly. Bake within 20 minutes until golden brown and a toothpick inserted in the center comes out clean.
5. Remove and allow the blondies to cool for 10 minutes before slicing into 15 bars. Wrap each bar in plastic wrap or place it in a resealable container.

Nutrition:

Calories: 125

Fat: 3g

Protein: 3g

Carbs: 23g

Blueberry-Zucchini Waffles

Preparation time: 15 minutes

Cooking time: 25 minutes

Servings: 4

Ingredients:

Nonstick cooking spray

- 1 cup unbleached all-purpose flour
- 1 cup whole-wheat pastry flour
- 2 teaspoons baking powder
- 1 teaspoon ground cinnamon
- ½ teaspoon salt
- 2 large eggs, beaten
- ¾ cup low-fat (1%) milk
- ¼ cup 100% pure maple syrup
- ½ cup unsweetened applesauce
- 2 tablespoons canola oil
- 1 medium zucchini, shredded
- 1 cup fresh or thawed frozen blueberries

Directions:

1. Preheat standard waffle iron and coat with cooking spray. Sift together the all-purpose flour, whole-wheat pastry flour, baking powder, cinnamon, and salt in a medium bowl.

2. Whisk the eggs, milk, maple syrup, applesauce, and oil in a separate medium bowl. Gently fold the dry fixings into the wet ingredients until just combined, being careful not to overmix. Gently fold in the zucchini and blueberries until incorporated.
3. Cook the waffles for about 6 minutes, or according to your waffle iron's instructions, using 1 cup of batter per waffle.
4. Transfer the cooked waffle to a plate, and repeat with the remaining batter to make a total of 4 waffles. Slice each waffle in half, and place one half in each of 8 resealable containers.

Nutrition:

Calories: 281

Fat: 7g

Protein: 8g

Carbs: 47g

Cranberry-Pistachio Granola with Yogurt

Preparation time: 15 minutes

Cooking time: 30 minutes

Servings: 5

Ingredients:

- 2 cups gluten-free rolled oats
- ½ cup unsalted shelled pistachios
- ½ cup dried cranberries
- ¼ teaspoon salt
- ½ cup honey
- ½ cup water, at room temperature
- 2½ cups nonfat plain Greek yogurt

Directions:

1. Preheat the oven to 350F. Line a sheet pan with parchment paper. Mix the oats, pistachios, and cranberries in a medium bowl. Sprinkle in the salt and stir to distribute evenly.

2. Whisk the honey plus water in a small bowl. Pour over the oat mixture and fold together to coat evenly. Allow sitting within 5 minutes to absorb the liquid.

3. Spread the oat batter evenly on the prepared sheet pan in a thin layer. Bake, stirring every 10 minutes within

30 minutes. Remove from the oven and let cool for 15 minutes.

4. Into each of 5 glass jars or containers, spoon ½ cup of yogurt and top with ¼ cup of granola.

Nutrition:

Calories: 184

Fat: 3g

Protein: 14g

Carbs: 26g

Quinoa and Berries Breakfast Bowl

Preparation time: 15 minutes

Cooking time: 15 minutes

Servings: 5

Ingredients:

- 1¼ cups quinoa
- 2½ cups low-fat (1%) milk
- ¼ cup 100% orange juice
- 1 tablespoon 100% pure maple syrup
- ½ teaspoon vanilla extract
- ¼ teaspoon ground cinnamon
- 1¼ cups fresh or thawed frozen blueberries
- 1¼ cups fresh strawberries, sliced

Directions:

1. Boil the quinoa and milk in a medium saucepan over high heat. Reduce the heat to low, cover, and simmer until all the liquid has been absorbed 12 to 15 minutes. Remove then fluff the quinoa with a fork.

2. In a medium bowl, whisk together the orange juice, maple syrup, vanilla, and cinnamon. Add the blueberries and strawberries, and toss to coat evenly.

3. Into each of 5 glass jars or containers, place ¾ cup of quinoa and top with 1/3 cup of berry mixture. Drizzle any extra sauce evenly into each jar.

Nutrition:

Calories: 257

Fat: 4g

Protein: 11g

Carbs: 45g

Tropical Parfait

Preparation time: 15 minutes

Cooking time: 20 minutes

Servings: 5

Ingredients:

- ½ cup plus 2 tablespoons unsweetened coconut flakes, divided
- ½ cup raw unsalted cashews, chopped
- ¼ cup 100% orange juice
- ¼ cup 100% pure maple syrup
- ½ teaspoon vanilla extract
- ½ teaspoon ground cinnamon
- 2 cups fresh or frozen and thawed pineapple chunks
- 2 cups fresh or frozen and thawed mango chunks
- 3¾ cups nonfat plain Greek yogurt

Directions:

1. Toast the coconut flakes until fragrant and slightly browned, about 3 minutes in a large saucepan over medium-low heat. Transfer the coconut flakes to a medium bowl and set aside to cool slightly. Use a paper towel to wipe out the saucepan.
2. In the same saucepan over medium-low heat, toast the cashews until fragrant and slightly browned about 4 minutes. Transfer the cashews to a small dish and set

aside to cool slightly. Use a paper towel to wipe out the saucepan.

3. Whisk the orange juice, maple syrup, vanilla, and cinnamon in a large bowl. Add the pineapple and mango, and toss to coat evenly.

4. Put the pineapple-mango mixture into the saucepan and bring to a boil. Reduce the heat and simmer until the pineapple and mango soften, and the liquid is reduced half, about 10 minutes.

5. Remove the saucepan and set aside to cool. Add the yogurt to the bowl with the toasted coconut, and toss to distribute evenly.

6. For the parfaits, into each of 5 glass jars, spoon ¾ cup of yogurt, top with 2/3 cup of fruit mixture (with the juices), and sprinkle with 1½ tablespoons of toasted cashews.

Nutrition:

Calories: 351

Fat: 12g

Protein: 21g

Carbs: 43g

Make-Ahead Cottage Cheese and Fruit Bowl

Preparation time: 15 minutes

Cooking time: 0 minutes

Servings: 5

Ingredients:

- 2½ cups low-fat cottage cheese
- 1¼ cups seedless green or red grapes halved
- 2½ cups diced cantaloupe
- 5 tablespoons unsalted sunflower seeds

Directions:

1. Into each of 5 containers or glass jars, spoon ½ cup of cottage cheese. Top with ¼ cup of seedless grapes, ½ cup of cantaloupe, and 1 tablespoon of sunflower seeds. Put airtight containers in the refrigerator for up to 5 days.

Nutrition:

Calories: 170

Fat: 5g

Protein: 16g

Carbs: 15g

Peanut Butter–Banana Oatmeal

Preparation time: 15 minutes

Cooking time: 5 minutes

Servings: 5

Ingredients:

- 2½ cups gluten-free quick-cooking oats
- 2½ cups skim milk
- 2½ cups water
- 3 tablespoons smooth peanut butter
- 3 tablespoons 100% pure maple syrup
- 1 teaspoon ground cinnamon
- ½ teaspoon vanilla extract
- 2 medium bananas, thinly sliced

Directions:

1. Mix the oats, milk, plus water in a saucepan over medium-low heat. Bring to a simmer, stirring frequently.
2. Cook until the oats begin to soften and the liquid thickens about 5 minutes. Remove the pan from the heat. Stir in the peanut butter, maple syrup, cinnamon, and vanilla until evenly distributed.
3. Divide the sliced bananas among 5 containers, then top each with 1 cup of cooled oatmeal. Put the airtight containers in the refrigerator for up to 5 days.

4. To reheat, microwave uncovered on high for 1 minute. Stir before eating and add a splash of milk, if desired.

Nutrition:

Calories: 333

Fat: 8g

Protein: 12g

Carbs: 55g

Banana-Strawberry Oatmeal Cups

Preparation time: 15 minutes

Cooking time: 50 minutes

Servings: 12

Ingredients:

- Nonstick cooking spray
- 3 cups gluten-free old-fashioned oats
- 1 teaspoon baking powder
- 1 teaspoon ground cinnamon
- ½ teaspoon salt
- 2 large eggs, beaten
- 1½ cups low-fat (1%) milk
- 1 medium banana, mashed
- ¼ cup 100% pure maple syrup
- 2 tablespoons unsalted butter, melted
- 1 teaspoon vanilla extract
- 1 cup sliced strawberries (about 8 medium)

Directions:

1. Preheat the oven to 350F. Line a 12-cup muffin tin and coat with cooking spray. Mix the oats, baking powder, cinnamon, and salt in a medium bowl.
2. Whisk the eggs, milk, banana, maple syrup, butter, and vanilla in a large bowl. Mix the dry fixing into the wet

ingredients until well combined. Fold in the sliced strawberries until evenly distributed.

3. Using a ¼-cup scoop, distribute the batter among the 12 muffin cups. Tap it a few times on your countertop to release any air bubbles.
4. Bake for 45 to 50 minutes until the edges of the oatmeal cups are slightly browned.
5. Remove and set aside to cool for 15 minutes, then transfer to a wire rack to continue cooling. Place the cooled muffins in a resealable container.

Nutrition:

Calories: 298

Fat: 9g

Protein: 10g

Carbs: 46g

Triple Berry Oatmeal-Almond Bake

Preparation time: 15 minutes

Cooking time: 60 minutes

Servings: 8

Ingredients:

- Nonstick cooking spray
- 1¾ cups gluten-free old-fashioned rolled oats
- ¼ cup almonds, chopped
- 2 teaspoons baking powder
- 1 teaspoon ground cinnamon
- ½ teaspoon salt
- 1½ cups low-fat (1%) milk
- ½ cup honey
- 1 large egg, beaten
- 1 teaspoon vanilla extract
- 2/3 cup fresh/thawed frozen blueberries
- 2/3 cup fresh/thawed frozen blackberries
- 2/3 cup fresh/thawed frozen raspberries

Directions:

1. Preheat the oven to 350F. Coat an 8-by-11.5-inch baking dish with cooking spray. Mix the oats, almonds, baking powder, cinnamon, and salt in a medium bowl.

2. Whisk the milk, honey, egg, and vanilla in a separate medium bowl. Pour the dry fixings into the wet

ingredients, and gently stir until just combined. Fold in the berries until evenly distributed.

3. Put the batter into the prepared baking dish. Use a spatula or the back of a spoon to distribute the batter evenly. Bake for about 1 hour until slightly browned and a toothpick inserted into the center comes out clean.

4. Remove, then allow to cool for 15 minutes before cutting into 8 even slices. Place the individual portions into 8 resealable containers.

Nutrition:

Calories: 203

Fat: 5g

Protein: 6g

Carbs: 37g

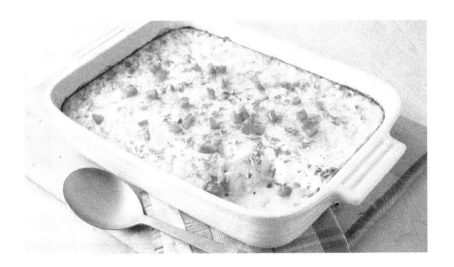

Veggie Delight Breakfast Egg Casserole

Preparation time: 15 minutes

Cooking time: 60 minutes

Servings: 6

Ingredients:

- Nonstick cooking spray
- ½ cup low-fat cottage cheese
- 8 large eggs
- 8 large egg whites
- 1 teaspoon Sriracha
- ½ teaspoon salt
- ¼ teaspoon freshly ground black pepper
- ½ cup shredded part-skim mozzarella cheese
- ¼ cup grated Parmesan cheese
- 1 cup cherry tomatoes, halved
- 3 medium carrots, peeled and shredded
- 1 medium zucchini, halved lengthwise and then cut into ½-inch half moons
- 1½ cups broccoli florets

Directions:

1. Preheat the oven to 350F. Coat an 8-by-11.5-inch baking dish with cooking spray.

2. In a blender, combine the cottage cheese, eggs, egg whites, Sriracha, salt, and pepper. Blend for 30 seconds to combine. Pour the egg batter into a large bowl.

3. Add the mozzarella and Parmesan to the egg mixture, and stir to incorporate. Add the tomatoes, carrots, zucchini, and broccoli, and toss to combine.

4. Put the batter into your baking dish, then bake, uncovered, for 55 minutes to 1 hour until the egg batter is set and a toothpick inserted into the center of the casserole comes out clean.

5. Remove the casserole, then allow to cool for 15 minutes before slicing into 6 pieces. Into each of 6 resealable containers, place a slice of casserole.

Nutrition:

Calories: 209

Fat: 10g

Protein: 21g

Carbs: 8g

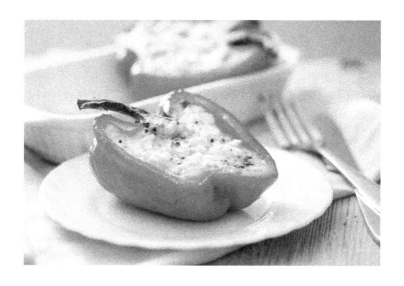

Egg and Spinach Stuffed Peppers

Preparation time: 15 minutes

Cooking time: 1 hour & 15 minutes

Servings: 5

Ingredients:

- Nonstick cooking spray
- 1 tablespoon olive oil
- 1 small onion, chopped
- 1 garlic clove, minced
- 4 ounces button mushrooms, chopped
- 3 ounces baby spinach (3 cups)
- 1 (14.5-ounce) can no-salt-added diced tomatoes
- ½ teaspoon salt, divided
- ¼ teaspoon freshly ground black pepper, divided
- 5 large eggs
- ½ cup low-fat (1%) milk
- 5 large red or green bell peppers
- 5 teaspoons grated Parmesan cheese

Directions:

1. Preheat the oven to 375F. Coat an 8-by-11.5-inch baking dish with cooking spray. In a medium skillet over medium heat, heat the oil.

2. Put the onion and garlic, and cook until the onion softens and the garlic is fragrant about 3 minutes. Put

the mushrooms and continue cooking until they soften about 5 minutes.

3. Add the spinach and cook until wilted, about 5 minutes. Add the diced tomatoes, ¼ teaspoon of salt, and 1/8 teaspoon of pepper and boil.
4. Reduce the heat, then simmer until the flavors combine, about 3 minutes. Remove the skillet from the heat and allow it to cool slightly.
5. Whisk the eggs, milk, and remaining ¼ teaspoon of salt and 1/8 teaspoon of pepper in a medium bowl.
6. Slice the tops off the peppers and trim the bottoms, so they stand without tilting. Using a paring knife, remove the membranes and seeds from inside each pepper.
7. Scoop ¼ cup of the vegetable mixture into each of the 5 peppers, and top each with 1 teaspoon of grated Parmesan. Then evenly distribute the egg batter among the 5 peppers.
8. Cover the peppers with aluminum foil, then bake for 50 minutes. Uncover and continue baking again within 10 minutes. Remove and set aside to cool slightly. Into each of 5 containers, place one stuffed pepper.

Nutrition:

Calories: 173

Fat: 9g

Protein: 11g

Carbs: 14g

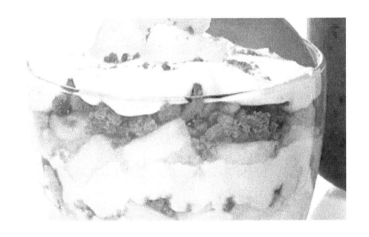

Pineapple Ginger Parfait

Preparation time: 15 minutes

Cooking time: 0 minutes

Servings: 6

Ingredients:

- 6 cups plain Greek yogurt
- 2 tablespoons grated fresh ginger
- 1 tablespoon honey
- 6 cups chopped pineapple
- ½ cup sliced almonds

Directions:

1. Mix the yogurt, ginger, and honey in a medium bowl.
2. Into each of 6 containers, place 1 cup of pineapple at the bottom, then top with 1 cup of yogurt mixture and a sprinkle of chopped almonds.
3. Store the airtight containers in the refrigerator for up to 5 days.

Nutrition:

Calories: 225

Fat: 4g

Protein: 18g

Carbs: 34g

Apple Nut Butter Quesadilla

Preparation time: 15 minutes

Cooking time: 0 minutes

Servings: 4

Ingredients:

- Per quesadilla (x4)
- 2 whole-wheat tortillas, divided
- 2 tablespoons almond butter, smooth or crunchy
- ½ apple, cut into ¼-inch slices
- 1 tablespoon hemp seeds
- Pinch ground cinnamon

Directions:

1. Put 1 tortilla on your cutting board and spread the almond butter onto the base. Place the apple slices onto the almond butter, then sprinkle with the hemp seeds and cinnamon.
2. Place the remaining tortilla on top, press down lightly, and cut into quarters. Repeat to create 3 additional quesadillas. Into each of 4 containers, place 1 quartered quesadilla. Store the airtight containers in the refrigerator for up to 3 days.

Nutrition:

Calories: 457

Fat: 26g

Protein: 17g

Carbs: 45g

Chocolate Cherry Oatmeal Cups

Preparation time: 15 minutes

Cooking time: 35 minutes

Servings: 12

Ingredients:

- Nonstick olive oil cooking spray
- 3 cups old-fashioned oats
- ¼ cup plus 1 tablespoon unsweetened cocoa powder
- ¼ cup chocolate protein powder
- 1 teaspoon baking powder
- ½ teaspoon salt
- 2 cups almond milk
- 2 cups halved cherries
- 2 large eggs, beaten
- 2 tablespoons coconut oil
- 2 tablespoons maple syrup

Directions:

1. Preheat the oven to 375°F. Oiled a 12-cup muffin tin with cooking spray. Mix the oats, cocoa powder, protein powder, baking powder, and salt in a large bowl. Mix well.

2. Add in the almond milk, cherries, eggs, coconut oil, and maple syrup. Stir together until well combined. Scoop

the mixture evenly into the muffin tin and bake for 30 to 35 minutes.

3. Remove the muffins from the cups and allow to cool before storing. Into each of 6 containers or eco-friendly sandwich bags, place 2 muffins. Store the airtight containers in the refrigerator for up to 5 days.

Nutrition:

Calories: 156

Fat: 6g

Protein: 7g

Carbs: 21g

Blueberry Fool Overnight Oats

Preparation time: 15 minutes

Cooking time: 0 minutes

Servings: 8

Ingredients:

- Per container (x8)
- 1 cup unsweetened dairy-free milk (soy, almond, oat)
- ½ cup old-fashioned oats
- Pinch salt
- 1 tablespoon plain yogurt (regular or Greek)
- ½ teaspoon grated lemon zest (4 teaspoons total)
- ¼ cup Blueberry Chia Jam (2 cups total)

Directions:

1. Gather 8 (16-ounce) jars or other prep containers. Into each jar, place the dairy-free milk, oats, and salt. Give this a quick stir.
2. Then add in the yogurt, lemon zest, and Blueberry Chia Jam; cover and place the jars in the refrigerator. Store the airtight containers in the refrigerator for up to 5 days.

Nutrition:

Calories: 300

Fat: 11g

Protein: 11g

Carbs: 40g

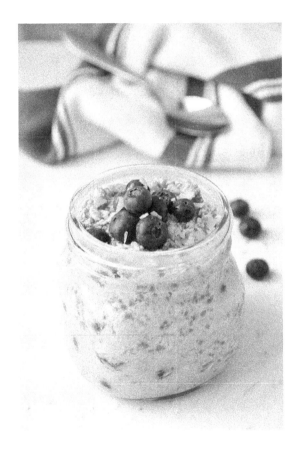

Zucchini Cheddar Scones

Preparation time: 15 minutes

Cooking time: 25 minutes

Servings: 8

Ingredients:

- 2½ cups all-purpose flour, plus 1 tablespoon
- ¼ cup granulated sugar
- 1½ teaspoons baking powder
- 1 teaspoon salt
- 1 teaspoon dried thyme
- ½ teaspoon baking soda
- 8 tablespoons (1 stick) cold unsalted butter, slice into tiny pieces
- ¾ cup low-fat milk
- 1 large egg
- 2 teaspoons white vinegar or lemon juice
- 1 cup shredded zucchini
- 1 cup shredded cheddar cheese, divided

Directions:

1. Preheat the oven to 400°F. Prepare 2 baking sheets with parchment paper, then set aside. In a large bowl, combine 2½ cups of flour, sugar, baking powder, salt, thyme, and baking soda and stir to combine.

2. Put the butter in the bowl and, using your hands, quickly work the butter into the flour batter until it resembles a coarse meal.

3. In a small bowl, combine the milk, egg, and vinegar, then add this to the flour and butter mixture.

4. Mix the shredded zucchini, ¾ cup of cheddar cheese, and the remaining 1 tablespoon of flour in a separate bowl. Toss to coat, then add this zucchini mixture to the dough and combine gently.

5. Pour the dough out onto a clean, lightly floured surface and gently work it into a round mound. Press it out into an 8-inch circle that is about ½ inch thick.

6. Cut it into 8 triangles and transfer each triangle to the lined baking sheets. Sprinkle the rest of the ¼ cup of cheddar cheese on top of the scones.

7. Bake within 20 to 25 minutes, or until the scones' tops are golden brown and a toothpick inserted in a scone comes out clean. Put in airtight containers in the fridge for up to 3 days.

Nutrition:

Calories: 355

Fat: 17g

Protein: 11g

Carbs: 40g

Good Morning Sweet Potato Jacket

Preparation time: 15 minutes

Cooking time: 15 minutes

Servings: 4

Ingredients:

- Per sweet potato jacket (x4)
- 1 small sweet potato
- ½ cup plain yogurt
- 2 tablespoons almond butter
- 3 tablespoons granola

Directions:

1. Poke each of your sweet potatoes several times with a fork and cook the sweet potatoes in the microwave until tender and the flesh is pierced easily with a fork, about 15 minutes. Let cool, then wrap each cooked potato in aluminum foil or store in a container or eco-friendly bag.
2. In a small container, combine the yogurt, almond butter, and granola and store them separately. Store the airtight containers in the refrigerator for up to 3 days.

Nutrition:

Calories: 426

Fat: 23g

Protein: 14g

Carbs: 45g

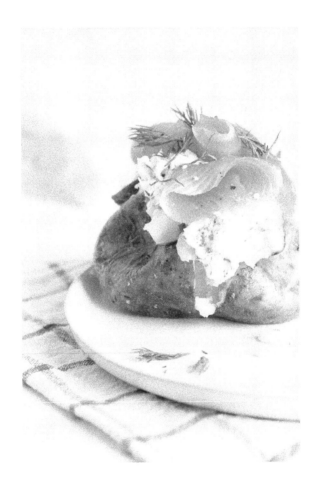

Strawberry Balsamic French Toast Bake

Preparation time: 15 minutes

Cooking time: 40 minutes

Servings: 6

Ingredients:

- Unsalted butter, for greasing
- 8 (1-inch-thick) slices brioche bread (stale or oven-dried), cut into 1-inch cubes, divided
- 4 ounces mascarpone
- 2 tablespoons powdered sugar
- 1 teaspoon vanilla extract
- 2 cups sliced or chopped strawberries, divided
- 4 large eggs
- 1 cup whole milk
- 1/3 cup brown sugar
- 2 tablespoons balsamic vinegar, plus more for serving

Directions:

1. Grease an 8-by-12-inch baking dish with butter or cooking spray. Place half of the cubed bread into the dish.
2. Mix the mascarpone, powdered sugar, and vanilla until smooth in a small bowl. Using a spoon, dollop this mixture on top of the bread and spread it out.

3. Top with 1 cup of strawberries, then the remaining cubed bread, and finish with the remaining 1 cup of strawberries.

4. Whisk the eggs, milk, brown sugar, and balsamic vinegar in a large bowl. Pour this mixture evenly over the bread. Push the mixture down so that the top layer of bread soaks up some of the custard.

5. Cover using aluminum foil or plastic wrap and let sit in the refrigerator for at least 1 hour—Preheat the oven to 350°F.

6. Remove the foil and bake within 30 to 40 minutes, until the top begins to brown. Remove, let cool, and divide into 6 equal squares. Drizzle with additional balsamic, if desired.

7. Into each of 6 containers, place 1 square. Put in your fridge for up to four days.

Nutrition:

Calories: 397

Fat: 23g

Protein: 9g

Carbs: 37g

Pumpkin Pancakes

Preparation time: 15 minutes

Cooking time: 25 minutes

Servings: 8

Ingredients:

- 2 cups buckwheat flour
- 2 cups canned pumpkin purée
- 2 cups low-fat milk or dairy-free milk
- 4 large eggs
- ¼ cup maple syrup
- 2 tablespoons melted coconut oil
- 2 teaspoons vanilla extract
- 2 tablespoons freshly squeezed lemon juice
- 1 teaspoon baking soda
- 1 teaspoon ground cinnamon
- ½ teaspoon ground nutmeg
- Butter, for greasing
- Maple syrup, for serving (optional)
- Nut butter, for serving (optional)
- Plain yogurt, for serving (optional)
- Apple compote, for serving (optional)

Directions:

1. In a blender, combine the buckwheat flour, pumpkin purée, milk, eggs, maple syrup, coconut oil, vanilla, lemon juice, baking soda, cinnamon nutmeg.
2. Blend on high within 30 seconds or until mixed well. If your blender cannot hold all the ingredients, whisk the ingredients in a large bowl.
3. Warm-up a nonstick skillet over medium heat and add a small amount of butter to grease the pan. Put 1/3 cup of batter onto the pan and cook until the edges start to puff up and look dry and the underside is lightly browned. Flip and cook within 30 to 60 more seconds. Repeat with the remaining batter.
4. If desired, serve with maple syrup, nut butter, yogurt, and apple compote. Put in airtight containers in the fridge for up to 3 days.

Nutrition:

Calories: 321

Fat: 14g

Protein: 12g

Carbs: 38g

Mushroom Asparagus Quiche with Quinoa Crust

Preparation time: 15 minutes

Cooking time: 1 hour & 25 minutes

Servings: 8

Ingredients:

For the quinoa:

- 1½ cups water
- ½ cup uncooked quinoa
- 1 tablespoon extra-virgin olive oil

For the crust:

- 2 large eggs
- ½ cup grated Parmesan cheese
- 2 teaspoons garlic powder
- 2 teaspoons onion powder
- 1 teaspoon dried thyme

For the filling:

- 2 tablespoons extra-virgin olive oil, divided
- 1 shallot, chopped
- 2 cups chopped asparagus
- 3 cups chopped cremini mushrooms
- 6 large eggs, beaten
- 1 cup crumbled goat cheese
- 1 teaspoon salt

- ½ teaspoon freshly ground black pepper

Directions:

1. Preheat the oven to 375°F. For the quinoa, boil the water, quinoa, and olive oil over high heat in a medium saucepot.

2. Adjust the heat to a simmer, cover, and cook until most of the water has been absorbed, about 15 minutes. Remove and let sit, covered, within 5 minutes.

3. Fluff your quinoa with a fork and cool to room temperature. For the crust, combine the eggs, Parmesan, garlic powder, onion powder, and thyme in a large bowl. Stir in the cooled quinoa.

4. Spread the crust mixture into an 11-inch tart pan or pie dish, pressing it into the bottom and the sides to create the crust edge. Bake for 15 minutes, until lightly browned. Remove and let cool 5 minutes.

5. For the filling, heat-up 1 tablespoon of olive oil over medium heat in a medium skillet. Put the shallot and sauté for 2 to 3 minutes.

6. Toss in the asparagus and cook for 5 minutes. Add in the mushrooms and the remaining 1 tablespoon of olive oil.

7. Sauté everything for another 5 to 7 minutes, until the asparagus has browned and the mushrooms have softened. Remove from the heat.

8. Mix the cooked vegetables with the beaten eggs, goat cheese, salt, and pepper in a large bowl. Pour this mixture into the prepared quinoa crust. Bake for 35 to 40 minutes until golden brown and set in the center.

9. Remove the finished quiche from the oven, let cool, and divide into 8 slices. Into each of 8 containers, place 1 slice of quiche. Store the airtight containers in the refrigerator for up to 4 days.

Nutrition:

Calories: 238

Fat: 15g

Protein: 14g

Carbs: 12g

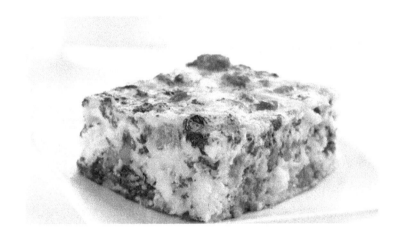

Italian Sausage Breakfast Bake

Preparation time: 15 minutes

Cooking time: 55 minutes

Servings: 6

Ingredients:

- 3 cups cubed Italian bread
- ¾ pound ground pork sausage, removed from casings
- 1 yellow bell pepper, chopped
- 1 red bell pepper, chopped
- ½ large yellow onion, thinly sliced
- 2 cups baby spinach
- 6 large eggs
- 1 cup low-fat milk
- ½ teaspoon fennel seed
- ½ teaspoon dried rosemary
- ¼ teaspoon freshly ground black pepper
- ¼ teaspoon salt

Directions:

1. Preheat the oven to 400°F. Oiled a 9-by-13-inch baking dish with cooking spray and set aside.
2. Lay the cubed bread on a baking sheet and coat with a light layer of cooking spray. Bake until the cubes begin to turn golden brown, 10 to 12 minutes. Remove from the oven and set aside in a large bowl.

3. Heat-up a medium skillet over high heat and spray lightly with cooking spray. Add the sausage and break it up, using a wooden spoon, until cooked for 5 to 7 minutes. Transfer the sausage to the bread bowl.
4. To the heated skillet, add the bell peppers and onion and cook for 7 to 8 minutes, until the onion starts to soften. In the end, add in the spinach so that it slightly wilts.
5. Add this mixture to the bread and sausage bowl and mix to combine. Transfer your batter to the baking dish.
6. Mix the eggs, milk, fennel, rosemary, pepper, and salt in a small bowl. Whisk the mixture well, and pour it over the baking dish. Use a spatula to press the mixture down gently.
7. Bake within 30 to 35 minutes until the liquid is set and the edges are bubbly. Remove from the oven, let cool, and cut into 6 squares.
8. Into each of 6 containers, place 1 baked square. Put in your fridge for up to 4 days.

Nutrition:

Calories: 265

Fat: 9g

Protein: 23g

Carbs: 24g

Bircher Muesli with Apple and Cinnamon

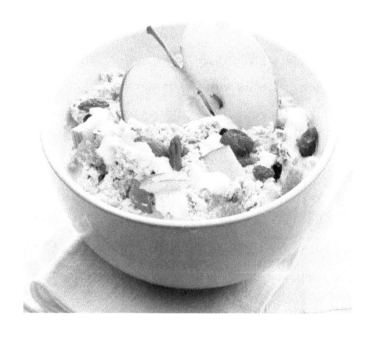

Preparation time: 15 minutes

Cooking time: 0 minutes

Servings: 4

Ingredients:

- 1 ½ cups wholegrain rolled oats
- 2 apples, skin on, grated
- 1 tsp. ground cinnamon
- 1 cup almond milk
- 1 cup plain, unsweetened yogurt

Directions:

1. Place the oats, grated apple, cinnamon, milk, and yogurt into a bowl and stir to combine. The mixture should be wet and reasonably thick, but it will depend on the yogurt brand you use.
2. Divide the mixture into your four containers or bowls, cover, and place in the fridge.
3. In the morning, simply grab it from the fridge and eat with a spoon! You'll love this cold, filling, and refreshing breakfast.

Nutrition:

Calories: 185

Fat: 3 g

Protein: 4 g

Carbs: 33 g

Prepped Fruit Salad with Lemon and Honey

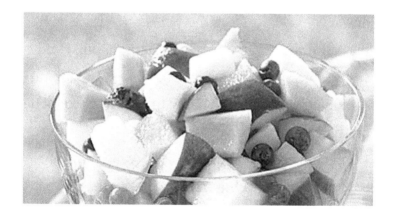

Preparation time: 15 minutes

Cooking time: 0 minutes

Servings: 3

Ingredients:

- 2 bananas, cut into chunks
- 4 large strawberries, cut into quarters
- 1 apple, core removed, flesh cut into small chunks
- 1 orange, cut into chunks
- 2 tbsp. honey
- 1 juicy lemon

Directions:

1. Place the bananas, strawberries, apple, orange, honey, and juice of one lemon in a bowl and stir to combine. Divide the fruit salad into your 3 containers, cover, and store in the fridge.
2. For extra protein, serve with plain Greek yogurt or a hard-boiled egg on the side.

Nutrition:

Calories: 176

Fat: 0 g

Protein: 2 g

Carbs: 46 g

Berry, Yogurt, and Chia Pots

Preparation time: 15 minutes

Cooking time: 0 minutes

Servings: 5

Ingredients:

- 2 cups mixed berries (frozen or fresh)
- 6 tbsp. chia seeds
- 1 cup (8floz) almond milk
- ½ cup (4floz) cold water
- 1 tsp. cinnamon
- 1 tsp. vanilla extract
- 1 cup (8floz) plain, unsweetened yogurt

Directions:

1. Divide the berries between your 5 pots or cups. Place the chia seeds, almond milk, water, cinnamon, and vanilla extract into a small bowl and stir to combine.
2. Divide the chia seed mixture between the 5 pots, and spoon on top of the berries. Divide the yogurt between the 5 pots and spoon on top of the chia mixture.
3. Put a bit of cinnamon over the yogurt and place an extra berry on top. Cover and place into the fridge.

Nutrition:

Calories: 139

Fat: 5 g

Protein: 4 g

Carbs: 17 g

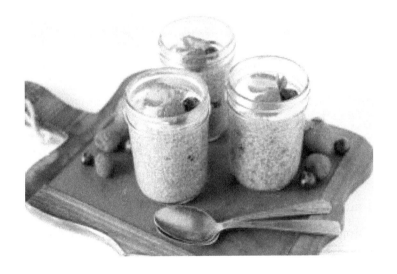

Salmon and Egg Muffins

Preparation time: 15 minutes

Cooking time: 8-10 minutes

Servings: 6

Ingredients:

- 4 eggs
- 1/3 cup milk
- Salt and pepper, to taste
- 1 ½ oz. smoked salmon, cut into small pieces
- 1 tbsp. finely chopped chives

Directions:

1. Preheat the oven to 356 degrees Fahrenheit and grease 6 muffin tin holes with a small butter. Place the eggs, milk, and a pinch of salt and pepper into a small bowl and lightly beat to combine.

2. Divide the egg batter between the 6 muffin holes, divide the salmon between the muffins and place it into each hole, and gently press down to submerge in the egg mixture.

3. Sprinkle each muffin with chopped chives and place in the oven for about 8-10 minutes or until just set. Leave to cool within 5 minutes before turning out and storing in an airtight container in the fridge.

Nutrition:

Calories: 93

Fat: 6 g

Protein: 8 g

Carbs: 1 g

Green Smoothie Freezer Packets

Preparation time: 15 minutes

Cooking time: 0 minutes

Servings: 7

Ingredients:

- 4 cups baby spinach leaves
- 2 cups chopped raw kale
- 1 avocado, flesh cut into chunks
- 2 green apples, skin on, cut into chunks
- 2 cups blueberries

Directions:

1. Place the spinach, kale, avocado, apples, and blueberries into a bowl and stir to combine. Divide the smoothie mixture between the 7 bags, seal, and place it into the freezer.
2. For the smoothie, place the contents of one smoothie packet into the blender, and add enough water to suit your preferred smoothie consistency, then store.

Nutrition:

Calories: 105

Fat: 3 g

Protein: 2 g

Carbs: 18 g

Soaked Oats with Vanilla, Dried Fruit, and Nuts

Preparation time: 15 minutes

Cooking time: 0 minutes

Servings: 4

Ingredients:

- 2 cups whole grain rolled oats
- 3 cups (24floz) almond milk
- 3 tsp. vanilla extract
- 4 prunes, chopped into small pieces
- 4 dates, chopped into small pieces
- 20 almonds, roughly chopped
- 12 walnuts, roughly chopped

Directions:

1. Place the oats, almond milk, vanilla extract, prunes, dates, almonds, and walnuts into a bowl and stir to combine. Divide the mixture into the 4 jars, seal or cover, then place into the fridge to soak overnight.

2. In the morning, if you find that the oats are a bit too stiff or dry, you can put a bit more almond milk to loosen it up.

Nutrition:

Calories: 300

Fat: 11 g

Protein: 9 g

Carbs: 41 g

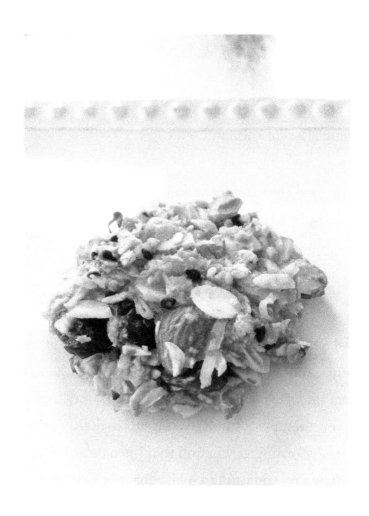

Toasted Granola Packs

Preparation time: 15 minutes

Cooking time: 7 minutes

Servings: 7

Ingredients:

- 2 tbsp. coconut oil
- 3 cups wholegrain rolled oats
- 4 tbsp. shredded coconut
- 3 tbsp. flaxseeds
- 3 tbsp. pumpkin seeds
- 3 tbsp. sunflower seeds
- 3 tbsp. chia seeds
- 10 dried apricots, chopped into small pieces
- 1 tsp cinnamon
- ¼ tsp. sea salt

Directions:

1. Warm coconut oil in a large pan or pot over medium heat. Add the oats, coconut, flaxseeds, pumpkin seeds, sunflower seeds, chia seeds, dried apricots, cinnamon, and sea salt; stir to combine.
2. Keep stirring the mixture as it gently toasts for about 7 minutes or until golden and aromatic. Leave in the pan to cool before filling your 7 bags or containers. Store in the pantry.

Nutrition:

Calories: 261

Fat: 11 g

Protein: 12 g

Carbs: 33 g

Date and Cocoa Oatmeal Mix

Preparation time: 15 minutes

Cooking time: 0 minutes

Servings: 7

Ingredients:

- 4 cups wholegrain rolled oats
- 1 tbsp. unsweetened cocoa powder
- 15 dates, chopped into small pieces
- Pinch of salt

Directions:

1. Place the oats, cocoa, dates, and salt into a bowl and stir to combine. Place into one large container or 7 small containers and store in the pantry.
2. To make the oatmeal, place one serving of dry mix into a pot and add 1 and ¼ cups (10fl oz.) of water or milk, stir, and simmer until thick.

Nutrition:

Calories: 191

Fat: 2 g

Protein: 7 g

Carbs: 37 g

Coconut and Almond Chia Pudding

Preparation time: 15 minutes

Cooking time: 0 minutes

Servings: 4

Ingredients:

- 6 tbsp. chia seeds
- 1 cup wholegrain rolled oats
- 4 tbsp desiccated coconut
- ½ tsp almond essence
- ½ tsp. vanilla extract
- 4 cups (32fl oz.) unsweetened coconut milk
- 32 raw almonds, roughly chopped

Directions:

1. Place the chia seeds, oats, desiccated coconut, almond essence, vanilla extract, coconut milk, and raw almonds into a bowl and stir to combine.
2. Divide between your 4 jars or containers, cover, and place in the fridge overnight.

Nutrition:

Calories: 296

Fat: 19 g

Protein: 10 g

Carbs: 24 g

Avocado, Kale, and Mixed Bean Bowls

Preparation time: 15 minutes

Cooking time: 10 minutes

Servings: 4

Ingredients:

- ½ onion, finely chopped
- ½ tsp paprika
- 1 fresh tomato, chopped into chunks
- 1 can (14 oz.) black beans, drained
- 1 can (14 oz.) kidney beans, drained
- Salt and pepper, to taste
- 2 avocadoes, flesh sliced
- 2 cups chopped kale

Directions:

1. Put a bit of olive oil into a pot and place over low heat; add the onions, paprika, tomato, black beans, and kidney beans and stir to combine.
2. Simmer over medium heat for 10 minutes until bubbling and thick, and add a pinch of salt and pepper to season.
3. Divide the bean mixture between your 4 bowls and leave to cool slightly before placing the sliced avocado and kale on top.

4. Put some extra olive oil over the top of the kale and avocado before covering plastic wrap and placing it into the fridge until needed.

Nutrition:

Calories: 290

Fat: 11 g

Protein: 12 g

Carbs: 38 g

Mango and Lime-Flavored Yogurt

Preparation time: 15 minutes

Cooking time: 0 minutes

Servings: 5

Ingredients:

- 2 mangoes, flesh removed and cut into small pieces
- 3 cups (24fl oz.) unsweetened Greek yogurt
- 1 tbsp. honey
- 1 lime

Directions:

1. Put half of the mango into a blender, use a stick blender, and blend to a pulp. Place the blended mango, remaining mango chunks, yogurt, honey, and grated zest of one lime into a bowl and stir to combine.
2. Divide into your 5 containers, cover, and store in the fridge. For an extra treat, sprinkle a few chopped almonds or some desiccated coconut on top before eating.

Nutrition:

Calories: 266

Fat: 14 g

Protein: 7 g

Carbs: 30 g

Pre-Made Banana Pancakes

Preparation time: 15 minutes

Cooking time: 0 minutes

Servings: 15

Ingredients:

- 2 large bananas, peeled & cut into chunks
- 3 eggs
- ½ cup ground almonds
- 1 tsp. vanilla extract
- ½ tsp baking powder
- Coconut oil, for frying

Directions:

1. Place the bananas, eggs, ground almonds, vanilla extract, and baking powder into a bowl and mash using a fork, handheld stick blender, or potato masher until smooth and combined.
2. Drizzle some coconut oil into a non-stick frying pan and place over medium heat until oil gets hot.
3. Place a scoop of pancake batter into the hot pan and cook on both sides until golden and cooked through. Place the cooked pancakes into your airtight container and store in the fridge.
4. Before eating the next morning, simply heat the pancakes in the microwave or on a dry, hot frying pan

until heated through. Serve with yogurt and fruit, or simply eat plain!

Nutrition:

Calories: 170

Fat: 11 g

Protein: 6 g

Carbs: 14 g

Spinach, Mushroom, and Feta Breakfast Pies

Preparation time: 15 minutes

Cooking time: 10 minutes

Servings: 8

Ingredients:

- 5 eggs
- 2 cups chopped spinach
- 1 cup sliced mushrooms (any kind)
- 2 oz. feta cheese, cut into small pieces/crumbled
- Salt and pepper, to taste

Directions:

1. Preheat the oven to 356 degrees Fahrenheit and grease a rectangular pie or casserole dish with butter. Place the eggs, spinach, mushrooms, feta, salt, and pepper into a bowl and whisk to combine.

2. Put the batter into your greased dish and place into the oven to bake for about 10 minutes until just set. Leave to cool before slicing into 8 pieces and placing them into an airtight container. Store in the fridge.

Nutrition:

Calories: 67

Fat: 5 g

Protein: 5 g

Carbs: 1 g

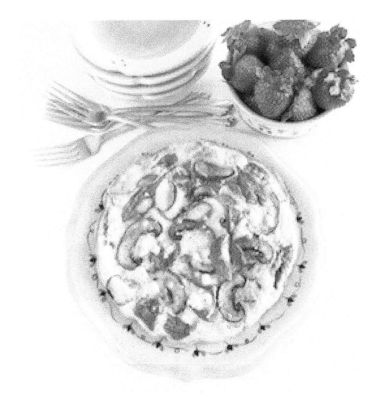

Bell Pepper and Bean Burritos

Preparation time: 15 minutes

Cooking time: 10 minutes

Servings: 4

Ingredients:

- 2 garlic cloves, finely chopped
- 2 red bell peppers, finely sliced
- 1 tsp. paprika
- ½ tsp. chili powder
- 1 can (14 oz.) black beans, drained
- Salt and pepper, to taste
- 2 eggs, lightly beaten
- 4 small flour or corn tortillas
- Fresh cilantro, chopped
- ½ fresh red chili, finely chopped

Directions:

1. Put some olive oil into your frying pan and place over medium heat. Add the garlic, bell peppers, paprika, chili powder, and sauté until the bell peppers are soft.

2. Add the black beans and a pinch of salt and pepper, stir to combine, continue to sauté. Push the bean and bell pepper mixture to one side of the pan and pour the lightly beaten eggs on the other side; stir them as they scramble until just cooked.

3. Turn off the heat and lay your tortillas on a board. Fill each tortilla with bell pepper, beans, and eggs. Sprinkle with cilantro and fresh chili, and tightly wrap. Carefully place the burritos into your container/s, cover, and put them into the fridge.

Nutrition:

Calories: 310

Fat: 8 g

Protein: 14 g

Carbs: 45 g

Chorizo and Sweet Potato Hash

Preparation time: 15 minutes

Cooking time: 15 minutes

Servings: 4

Ingredients:

- 3 cups sweet potato, cubed (about 2 large sweet potatoes)
- 1 chorizo sausage, sliced
- 1 cup spinach leaves, chopped
- 3 eggs, lightly beaten

Directions:

1. Put the sweet potatoes into a pot, cover with water, and place over medium heat until boiling. Leave to simmer, uncovered, until the sweet potatoes are soft but not mushy.

2. Drizzle some olive oil into a non-stick frying pan and place over medium heat. Place the chorizo into the hot frying pan and sauté for a few minutes until crispy and the oil has melted out.

3. Place the sweet potatoes into the frying pan and stir them as they sauté for a few minutes; it's okay if you crush them a bit. Put the spinach in the pan and stir into the sweet potatoes and chorizo until wilted.

4. Put the egg over the top of the sweet potato mixture and allow it to seep through the potatoes; make little holes

with a wooden spoon to let the egg combine with the other ingredients if you need to.

5. Cook the hash for a few minutes or until the egg has just set. Cut into 4 pieces and either store them in one large container or 4 single-serve containers.

6. Place into the fridge to store until needed. Eat hot or cold!

Nutrition:

Calories: 236

Fat: 11 g

Protein: 12 g

Carbs: 24 g

Blueberry and Mint Parfaits

Preparation time: 15 minutes

Cooking time: 0 minutes

Servings: 4

Ingredients:

- 1 ½ cups wholegrain rolled oats
- 1 cup (8fl oz.) almond milk
- 2 cups (16fl oz.) unsweetened Greek yogurt
- 1 cup fresh blueberries (can also use frozen, no need to thaw first)
- 4 small fresh mint leaves, finely chopped

Directions:

1. Place the oats and almond milk into a bowl and stir together to combine. Spoon the oat and almond milk mixture evenly into your 4 containers.
2. Place a drop of yogurt into each container on top of the oats. Divide half of the blueberries between the 4 containers and sprinkle on top of the yogurt.
3. Put another layer of yogurt, then another layer of blueberries. Sprinkle the fresh mint over the top of each parfait. Cover and place into the fridge to store until needed!

Nutrition:

Calories: 272

Fat: 8 g

Protein: 10 g

Carbs: 25 g

Peanut Butter and Banana Breakfast Cake

Preparation time: 15 minutes

Cooking time: 15 minutes

Servings: 8

Ingredients:

- 3 bananas, mashed
- 4 tbsp. natural peanut butter
- 3 eggs
- 1 cup almond flour
- 1 cup (8fl oz.) almond milk
- 1 tsp. baking powder
- 1 tsp. vanilla extract

Directions:

1. Preheat the oven to 356 degrees Fahrenheit and prepare a baking dish by lining it with baking paper.
2. Place the bananas, peanut butter, eggs, almond flour, almond milk, baking powder, and vanilla extract into a bowl and stir to combine.
3. Put the batter into the prepared baking dish, place it into the oven; bake for approximately 15 minutes, or just set.
4. Leave to cool before slicing into 8 pieces and storing in an airtight container in the fridge. Eat hot or cold!

Nutrition:

Calories: 200

Fat: 12 g

Protein: 7 g

Carbs: 16 g

Strawberry, Pumpkin Seed, and Coconut Oat Baked Crisp

Preparation time: 15 minutes

Cooking time: 15 minutes

Servings: 8

Ingredients:

- 3 tbsp. pumpkin seeds
- 2 cups wholegrain rolled oats
- ½ cup desiccated coconut
- 1 tsp. cinnamon
- 1 egg, lightly beaten
- 2 tbsp. honey
- ½ cup (4loz) almond milk
- ½ tsp. baking powder
- 1 cup fresh strawberries, stalks removed, cut into quarters

Directions:

1. Preheat the oven to 356 degrees Fahrenheit and prepare a baking tray by lining it with baking paper.
2. Place the pumpkin seeds, oats, coconut, cinnamon, egg, honey, almond milk, and baking powder into a bowl and stir to combine.

3. Press half of your batter into the lined tray, then place the strawberries over the top in an even layer. Press the rest of the oat mixture over top of the strawberries.
4. Place into the oven and bake within 15 minutes or until golden. Leave to cool before slicing into 8 pieces and storing in the fridge or freezer until needed!

Nutrition:

Calories: 160

Fat: 7 g

Protein: 7 g

Carbs: 19 g

Breakfast Tacos with Eggs, Bell Pepper and Mushrooms

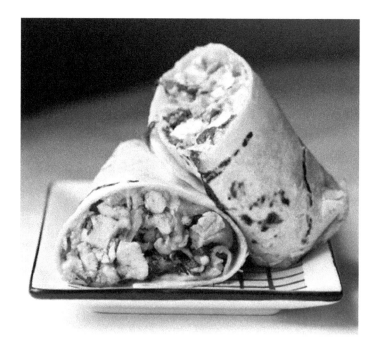

Preparation time: 15 minutes

Cooking time: 15 minutes

Servings: 8

Ingredients:

- 2 red bell peppers, core and seeds removed, flesh sliced
- 4 large Portobello mushrooms, sliced
- Salt and pepper, to taste
- 6 eggs, lightly beaten
- 8 whole meal tortilla wraps
- 4 tbsp. plain Greek yogurt
- 1 fresh red chili, finely chopped
- A handful of fresh cilantros, roughly chopped

Directions:

1. Put some olive oil into a pan and place over medium heat. Add the bell peppers, mushrooms, and a pinch of salt and pepper, sauté until soft.
2. Press your veggies to the side of the pan and pour the eggs on the other side, stirring and pushing them with a wooden spoon continuously as they scramble, cook until just set.
3. Remove and place your tortillas onto a large board or on a clean bench.
4. Spread a small amount of Greek yogurt onto each wrap, divide and put the bell peppers and mushrooms

between each wrap. Place on top of the yogurt, and then do the same with the egg between the wraps.

5. Finish with a sprinkle of chili and cilantro on top of each one! Carefully fold them up and place them in your chosen containers.

6. Place into the fridge until needed! These are best eaten cold due to the Greek yogurt addition.

Nutrition:

Calories: 387

Fat: 15 g

Protein: 22 g

Carbs: 47 g

Salmon, Kale, Ricotta and Egg Fry-pan Cake

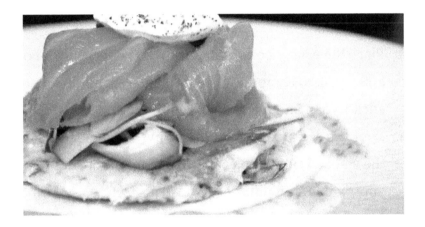

Preparation time: 15 minutes

Cooking time: 7 minutes

Servings: 6

Ingredients:

- 5 eggs, lightly beaten
- 4 oz. ricotta cheese
- 2 cups kale, finely sliced
- Salt and pepper, to taste
- 2 oz. smoked salmon, cut into small pieces

Directions:

1. Place the eggs, ricotta, kale, salt, and pepper into a bowl and whisk to combine. Drizzle some olive oil into a non-stick frypan and place over medium heat.
2. Pour the egg mixture into the frying pan and sprinkle the smoked salmon pieces over the top—Cook for approximately 7 minutes or until just set.
3. Leave to cool before slicing into 6 pieces and storing them in the fridge until needed!

Nutrition:

Calories: 120

Fat: 7 g

Protein: 11 g

Carbs: 2 g

Turkey and Artichokes Breakfast Casserole

Preparation time: 15 minutes

Cooking time: 60 minutes

Servings: 12

Ingredients:

- 1 1/2 pound ground turkey
- 2 green onion, sliced
- 1 medium green bell pepper, diced
- 14 ounces artichoke hearts, chopped
- 2 ½ cups fresh baby spinach
- 1/2 of a medium onion, peeled, diced
- 1/2 teaspoon cumin
- ¾ teaspoon ground black pepper
- 1/2 teaspoon oregano
- 1 teaspoon salt
- 1 teaspoon red chili powder
- 2 tablespoons avocado oil
- 16 eggs, beaten

Directions:

1. Switch on the oven, then set it to 375 degrees F and let preheat. Meanwhile, take a skillet pan, place it over medium heat, add oil, and when hot, add onion and green bell pepper.

2. Then add turkey, season with cumin, black pepper, oregano, salt, and red chili powder, stir well and cook for 10 minutes until meat is thoroughly cooked and nicely browned.
3. Add 2 cups spinach into cooked meat, stir well and continue cooking for 2 minutes until spinach leaves have wilted.
4. Take a 9 by 13 inches casserole dish or twelve oven safe meal prep glass containers, spoon in the turkey-spinach mixture, spread it evenly, and then top with artichokes.
5. Beat the eggs, pour it over artichokes in the casserole, and then sprinkle with green onion and remaining spinach and bake the casserole for 45 minutes until thoroughly cooked.
6. For meal prepping, let casseroles or containers cool completely, cover the casserole well with aluminum foil or close the containers with a lid, and store in the refrigerator for up to five days or freeze for three months. Reheat the casserole in the microwave until hot and serve.

Nutrition:
Calories: 184.7
Fat: 11.7 g
Carbs: 6.2 g
Protein: 13.9 g

Granola

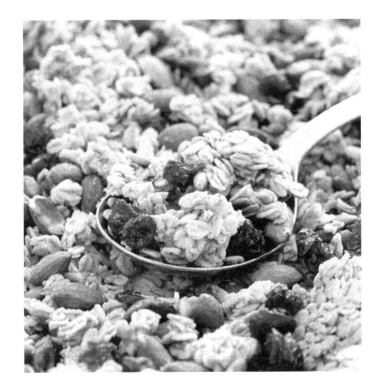

Preparation time: 10 minutes

Cooking time: 20 minutes

Servings: 10

Ingredients:

- 1 cup raisins
- 3 cups rolled oats, old-fashioned
- 1 cup sliced almonds
- 1/2 teaspoon ground cinnamon
- 1/2 teaspoon salt
- 1/2 cup honey
- 1/2 cup olive oil

Directions:

1. Switch on the oven, then set it to 300 degrees F, then place the baking rack in the middle of the oven and let preheat.
2. Place oil in a large bowl, whisk in cinnamon, salt, and honey until combined, then add almonds and oats and stir until well coated.
3. Take a rimmed baking sheet, line it with parchment paper, spoon oats mixture on it, then bake within 20 minutes until granola is golden brown, stirring halfway through.
4. Sprinkle raisins on top of granola, press it lightly and then let the granola cool.

5. Break granola into small pieces, then transfer granola into an airtight container and store for up to one month at room temperature.
6. When ready to eat, add some of the granola in a bowl, pour in milk, top with berries, and serve.

Nutrition:

Calories: 322

Fat: 17.1 g

Carbs: 40.5 g

Protein: 5.7 g

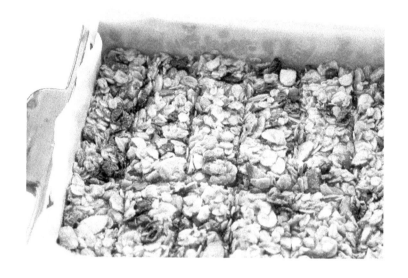

Almond Cranberry Chocolate Granola Bars

Preparation time: 20 minutes

Cooking time: 25 minutes

Servings: 12

Ingredients:

- 1 1/2 cups rolled oats, old-fashioned
- 1/4 cup chocolate chips
- 3/4 cup sliced almonds
- 1/3 cup cranberries, dried
- 1/3 cup honey
- 1/8 teaspoon salt
- 2 tablespoons brown sugar
- 3 tablespoons butter, unsalted
- 1/2 teaspoon vanilla extract, unsweetened
- 2 tablespoons peanut butter

Directions:

1. Switch on the oven, then set it to 325 degrees and let preheat. Take a medium saucepan, place it over medium-low heat, add the butter, honey, sugar, salt, and vanilla, stir well until combined, and cook for 5 minutes until the sugar has dissolved and the butter has melted.

2. Meanwhile, place oats in a medium bowl, add almonds, and stir until mixed. Pour in prepared honey mixture, stir until well combined, and let the mixture stand at room temperature for 10 minutes.

3. Then add chocolate chips and cranberries and fold until just mixed. Take a 9 by 9 inches casserole dish, line it with a parchment sheet, spoon in prepared oats mixture, spread and firmly press into the pan by using the back of a glass, and bake for 25 minutes until crunchy.

4. Let it cool, then cut into twelve bars, then put in an airtight container for up to 1 week or fridge for up to one month.

Nutrition:

Calories: 190

Fat: 13 g

Carbs: 18 g

Protein: 4 g

Cinnamon Raisin Granola

Preparation time: 10 minutes

Cooking time: 30 minutes

Servings: 5

Ingredients:

- 1 cup shredded coconut, unsweetened
- 1/2 cup raisins
- 1 cup pumpkin seeds
- 1/2 cup chopped pecans
- 1 cup sunflower seeds
- 1/2 cup sliced almonds
- 1/4 teaspoon salt
- 1/2 teaspoon allspice
- 1 tablespoon cinnamon
- 1 teaspoon vanilla extract, unsweetened
- 2 tablespoons maple syrup
- 1/3 cup coconut oil
- 1/4 cup honey

Directions:

1. Switch on the oven, then set it to 300 degrees F and let it preheat. Meanwhile, place all the ingredients in a large bowl, except for vanilla, maple syrup, oil, and honey, and stir until well mixed.

2. Put vanilla, maple syrup, oil, and honey stir well in a saucepan over low heat and cook for 5 minutes until melted.

3. Meanwhile, take a 10 by 15 inches baking sheet and then line it with parchment paper. Pour this mixture over granola mixture in the bowl and mix by hand until combined.

4. Transfer granola mixture onto the prepared baking sheet spread it evenly, and bake for 25 minutes until golden brown, stirring halfway through.

5. Cool the granola on a wire rack and then break it into small pieces. Transfer granola into an airtight container and then store for up to one month at room temperature.

6. When ready to eat, add some of the granola in a bowl, pour in milk, top with berries, and serve.

Nutrition:

Calories: 129.2

Fat: 1 g

Carbs: 31 g

Protein: 1 g

CPSIA information can be obtained
at www.ICGtesting.com
Printed in the USA
BVHW040610080321
601991BV00008B/523